Negative Calorie Diet with Smart Fat Guide

LELA GIBSON

CONTENTS

Negative Calorie Diet

Cookbook & Guide Which Will Help You To Burn Body Fat, Lose Weight And Live Healthy

Lela Gibson

Introduction

I would like to thank you for buying the book, "Negative Calorie Diet".

This book contains proven steps and strategies on how to burn body fat, lose weight and eat healthy.

Are you on the verge of giving up on your weight loss goals? Have you tried reducing your fat intake, eating fewer carbohydrates and all the diets that call for eating fewer proteins and carbohydrates, drank a lot of water, but you don't lose any weight? Does nothing seem to work?Well, I guess losing hope is understandable, but wait, DO NOT GIVE UP JUST YET! There is one more option, the best option in fact: The Negative Calorie Diet.

If we are to go by the facts, theNegative Calorie Diet is the fastest way to lose weight; you can lose up to 14 pounds a week when you adopt the diet! Thanks to this diet, losing weight is no longer a random dream or a hope; it is a reality for thousands of people across the globe.

In this book, you will learn more about the Negative Calorie Diet, how it works and some amazing recipes that will help you burn fat.

Thanks again for buying this book, I hope you enjoy it!

Negative Calorie Diet: What Is It

This unique diet draws upon theidea that some foodshave the 'negative calorie' effect that we ought to consider in burning fat. A food is considered to have a negative calorie effect when the calories these foods use to digest are typically higherthan the calories in the foods themselves.

When you eat something, you begin by chewing, a process that consumes energy. Some foods such as those higher in stringy fibers like celery will require more chewing, which will result in more energy expenditure, and there are otherslike pasta and cakes that don't require as much chewing.

After chewing, the foods go to the stomach through the esophagus and the other processes of digestion take over until absorption takes place and the body excretes the residual mass.

With negative calorie foods, this entire process uses up more calories than the foods have. The extra calories the body has to provide in order to process the foods are taken from the fat stores, and the more of these negative calorie foods you eat, the more your fat stores will lose calories, and as a result, the more fatyou will lose.

Let us take broccoli as an example: 100 grams (contains 25 calories).

When you eat 100 grams of broccoli, it takes your body about 80 calories worth of energy to digest it. This results in a net calorie use of 55 calories that should come from the fat stores in your body. As you can see, the 55 calories make up the negative net calorie.

Let us now take a counter example of a piece of cake containing 400 calories.

Your body will take about 150 calories to digest the piece of cake, leaving net 250 caloriesdeposited in the body and stored as fat.

The negative calorie diet consists of over 100 foods proven to have negative calorie qualities. Most of these foods are fruits and veggies that are high in fiber. Let us look at them in more detail in the following chapter.

Negative Calorie Food List

Here is a list of negative calorie foods:

Vegetables

Vegetables are highly nutritious and not high in calories when compared to many processed foods. Nonetheless, some vegetables are superior especially when it comes to the negative calorie food list. The following are vegetables you should consider including in your diet.

Artichokes	Bean sprouts	Broccoli	Cabbage	Cauliflower
Asparagus	Beets and beet greens	Brussels sprouts	Carrots	Celery
Chives	Cucumbers	Green beans	Mushrooms	Peppers (red, green, yellow)
Pumpkin	Sauerkraut	Spinach	String beans	Turnips
Corn	Eggplant	Lettuce	Peas	Pickles
Radishes	Scallions	Squash	Tomatoes	Zucchini
Garlic	Onion	Watercress		

Fruits

Just like vegetables, fruits are a healthier option and always the recommended healthy alternative to sugary foods. It is therefore a better idea to snack on a bunch of grapes than it is to snack on candy.

However, when it comes to fruit choices, you also need to make better choices because some fruits are high in calories; thus, not providing you the negative calorie effect you are looking for in negative calorie foods

The list below contains some good negative-calorie fruits you can eat:

Apples	Blackberries	Cantaloupe	Cranberries	Grapefruit
Honeydew melon	Lemons	Mangoes	Apricots	Blueberries
Cherries	Currants	Grapes	Kiwi	Limes
Nectarines	Oranges	Pears	Pomegranates	Strawberries
Watermelon	Peaches	Pineapple	Raspberries	Tangerines
Prunes				

Herbs and Spices

When it is a question of what you eat, even herbs and spices
matter. Below is a complete list of herbs and spices you should
always go for.

Chili pepper	Cloves	Ginger	Parsley	Cinnamon
Mustard seeds	Cayenne	Anise	Coriander/ Cilantro	Dill
Cumin	Fennel seeds			

Meat, Fish and Seafood

Red meat can be harmful to you, and many negative calorie diets don't recommend it; however, you do not have to avoid eating meat altogether, as it provides essential proteins and other nutrients. A good source of protein is fish for instance. Fish is lower in calories but high in essential nutrients like omega-3 fatty acids.

If you are allergic to fish, or if you are not a big fan of it, you can alternatively include small/reasonable potions of meat and chicken in your diet (I will teach you how in the recipes section).

The table below shows some of the best fish and seafood to include in your diet:

Clams	Crayfish	Mussels	Shrimp	Crab
Flounder	Tuna	Abalone	Buffalo fish	Cod
Terrapin	Bass	Catfish	Trout	

How To Make The Transition To Negative Calorie Diet

Now that you know what to eat, let us see exactly how you are going to be eating all that.

1. Make a smooth transition into the negative calorie diet so that you are comfortable with the entire process. Start by adding some negative calorie foods to the foods you normally eat in every meal in the 1:1 ratio. For instance, if having pasta with meatballs, you can serve 50% of this food and add chunks of zucchini to fill the other half.

You can also add a mixed salad to each meal you have; the salad should comprise of not less than 90% negative calorie foods. This means you have to look for ways to substitute any unwanted content such as any creamy high-fat substances with something like raspberry vinaigrette.

After some time, start slowly substituting the foods with the good (negative calorie) ones until your plate contains up to 90% negative calorie foods.

Note: We are only adding vegetables and fruits so far, not necessarily fully prepared negative calorie meals. Next, we will discuss the recipes so that you have entirely cooked meals too.

2.Use several vegetables to make a stir-fry. You can also make smoothie shakes with your favorite fruits including some berries. As said before, the negative calorie diet is largely a fruits and vegetables diet. However, this does not mean you should now start worrying about how you will survive as a vegetarian.

You can occasionallyenjoy small servings of chicken and some meat, and the recipes in the following chapter will reflect that. Nonetheless, the meats have to be in small amounts; remember, you are losing weight and so, you have to make some sacrifices.

First Thing to Do

Buy all the foods you think you require from the list, wash, cut them into bits then store them in airtight containers for storage (in the fridge) so that you will have them handy anytime you need them. You do not want to come home from work tired in the evening without having a bunch of these foods readily available. If you do, you will be extremely tempted to grab something unhealthy.

If you are wondering whether you will be hungry on this diet plan, just know that you will not because these foods are filling because they are high in fiber as well as water; the perfect combination to be full.

Second Thing to Do

Once you have identified the foods you want to eat, the next step is to actually get rid of the foods you want to stay away from. Let's face it, many times you end up eating some foods, not because you're hungry, but simply because you've seen them. High calorie foods often tend to be appetizing and inviting. Macronutrients such as carbohydrates work to stimulate the brain's pleasure center. This means you end up craving high carb foods and overeating in order to keep getting that 'comfort' they provide. Unfortunately, such foods are quite high in calories. Therefore, they ensure that your body has more than enough calories to store up. This is why you need to do a kitchen sweep.

Start by checking your list and determining which foods need to go. If you've not fully transitioned to the negative calorie diet, you need to determine which foods you'll get rid of first and which ones you'll get rid of later. Write down a list so that you can check your progress. For example, you may start by getting rid of pasta and red meat. Next, you can get rid of alcoholic drinks and high calorie fruits.

The idea is to gradually get rid of those foods that are high in calories. This will leave you with foods that will help you achieve your goal on the negative calorie diet. Once you've done that, you can move on to the next step.

Note: While on this diet, you should have no room for alcohol, sugar, or any sugar substitutes except stevia simply because sugar intake causes your body to produce more insulin. This hormone signals/tells the fat cells to pick up and convert any excess glucose into fat. Therefore, eating more sugar means more production of insulin and consequently, more deposits in the fat cells. We are trying to reduce fat in your body, not create more of it. In this regard, avoid all commercial dressings since most of them contain sugar and high fat content.

Third Thing to Do

It's well and good to know which foods to eat when you're on the negative calorie diet but it's another thing to make a meal out of the various foods. This is why the third step is to embrace meal planning.

You can plan for breakfast, lunch, dinner and snacks. Start by asking yourself what you want to eat during such meals. For example, you may plan to eat salads for lunch. As you have read, you can actually include many negative calorie foods in salads. This means that you can create various types of salads to eat throughout the week. Take some time to think of the combinations of foods you'd want to eat. This will keep the diet fresh and interesting.

Meal planning also enables you to know what foods to buy for the week. Remember, you'll be eating a lot of fruits and vegetables. These types of foods tend to taste better when they are fresh. Unfortunately, they also tend to go bad fast. This means you'll have to plan your shopping well in order to get the best out of the foods. If you know what you'll be eating, you'll purchase whatever is needed and this will enhance your experience as you continue your diet.

Now that we have that out of the way, let us start cooking!

Negative Calorie Diet Recipes

While on a strict diet (such as this one), you might have a problem trying to decide what kind of dressing to use for your meals. Since I know it is important to be careful about what you are using, I will start by giving you two simple dressings that you will use on any meal you want.

Garlic and Herbs Dressing

Mix 1/2 cup of cold-pressed extra-virgin olive oil with juice from 1 lemon, 2 crushed garlic cloves and ¼ cup apple cider vinegar. Add some of your favorite negative caloriedried herbs such as parsley and cilantro.

This will yield 1 cup of dressing. Store the dressing in the fridge (for up to one month) to use on your foods.

Dijon and Yoghurt Dressing

For a delicious vegetable dip, mix Dijon mustard (2 tablespoons) with 2 cups low-fat yoghurt then add a pinch of chili pepper and a teaspoon of mixed dried herbs to spice it up.

Breakfast Recipes

Pumpkin Pancakes

Serves 4

Ingredients

1 cup of canned pumpkin

1 1/4 cups of water

2 teaspoons of cinnamon

2 cups Krusteaz pancake mix

1 egg, slightly beaten

1 teaspoon of baking powder

For the topping

1/4 cup of sliced pecans

5 tablespoons of pure maple syrup

Instructions

Combine all the ingredients for the pancake batter.

On a griddle or pan over medium heat sprayed with a little cooking spray, create a 10 cm circle of batter.

When the pancakes turn brown at the edges and you notice even bubbling across the top, flip them over to cook the other side.

In the meantime, toast pecans in a small pan until they turn slightly brown and give out the fragrance.

Serve with heated pure maple syrup.

Apple and Cinnamon with Almonds and Oat Bran

Serves 4

Ingredients

4 large apples

1 teaspoon of ground cinnamon

1/4 cup of oat bran

10 almonds, toasted and chopped

1 teaspoon of unrefined coconut oil

2 cups of unsweetened vanilla almond milk

2 packets monk fruit extract

Instructions

Wash the apples and cut into cubes.

Melt the coconut oil in a large nonstick skillet over medium high heat. Add the cinnamon and apples then cook for 2-3 minutes until the apples soften.

Remove from the heat, add almond milk, stir in the monk fruit extract and oat bran. Once mixed return back to the heat, stir, and bring to a simmer.

Cook for about one minute, until the mixture becomes thick and creamy.

Divide the mixture among four bowls then sprinkle each one with toasted almonds.

Negative Calorie Smoothie

Serves 2

Ingredients

5 strawberries

½ medium papaya

1 grapefruit

¼ cup ice

Instructions

Put all the ingredients in a blender; blend until smooth.

Serve and garnish with some strawberries and enjoy.

Lunch Recipes

Vegetable Soup

Serves 6

This is not your regular veggie soup; yes, it is simple, but it is full of negative calorie foods only.

Ingredients

6 cups of vegetable stock

1 cup of celery, diced

1 cup of green beans cut into about 1 inch pieces

1 medium zucchini, diced (approximately 2 cups)

1 cup small turnip, diced

1 jalapeno, seeded and finely chopped

1 medium onion, diced

1 cup of cauliflower florets

2 cups of shredded cabbage

3 cloves of garlic, finely chopped

2 cups of baby spinach

Salt and pepper to taste

Instructions

Mix the ingredients (except the spinach) in a pot, and bring to a boil.

Cover and let it simmer for 20 minutes.

Add the spinach, stir, and let it cook for one more minute.

Remove from the heat and serve.

Toast with Tomatoes

Serves 4

Ingredients

8 cups of spinach

½ ripe avocado, mashed well with a fork

Salt to taste

Freshly ground black pepper to taste

4 slices of natural gluten-free bread

4 (½-inch) slices ripe tomato

4 eggs, poached

Green hot sauce

Instructions

Place a nonstick skillet over medium high heat.

Add the spinach and cook until it wilts. Move the spinach to a colander and strain out as much water as possible. Put the now drained spinach in a bowl and season with green hot sauce and salt.

Use a toaster to toast the bread then season the avocado with salt. Evenly spreadthe pieces of avocado over each piece of toast then add a slice of tomato on top. Use pepper and salt to season the tomatoes and use the spinach mixture to top each slice evenly.

Place every piece of toast on a fresh plate. Finally, top with a poached egg and serve.

Meatballs with Mushroom Gravy

Serves 4

Ingredients

12 ounces lean ground beef

1 ounce Parmigiano Reggiano cheese, finely chopped

2 tablespoons arrowroot, dissolved in 2 teaspoons of stock

8 cups washed spinach

1 cup thinly sliced onion

4 cups sliced cremini mushrooms

Olive oil cooking spray

Freshly ground black pepper

Salt to taste

4 cups unsalted beef stock

1 cup finely chopped puffed brown rice

Instructions

Put the beef in a large bowl and push it to one side. Add rice and a cup of the stock to the other side of the mixing bowl; season with pepper and salt and allow the rice to absorb the stock for about 1 minute.

Mix the beef and rice using an electric hand mixture until well mixed. Taste and adjust the seasoning then use the mixture to form 16 meatballs.

Coat a skillet with olive oil cooking spray and place over medium heat. Once hot, put the meatballs and brown for one minute on one side. Turn and brown the opposite side for around 30 seconds and transfer to a plate.

Add the mushrooms to the skillet and sauté for a few minutes. Add the meatballs back to the skillet, then add the beef stock, arrowroot mixture, and cook until meatballs are cooked through.

Add the spinach and season with pepper and salt and cook until the spinach is wilted. Add the cheese, stir, and serve.

Dinner Recipes

Brussels Sprouts with Lemon and Almond Dressing

Serves 3-4

Ingredients

3 pints Brussels sprouts, shaved thinly

5 teaspoons of freshly minced garlic

Crushed red pepper flakes

1/2 cup of chopped fresh flat-leaf parsley

Salt

1 1/2 teaspoons of extra-virgin olive oil

1/4 cup of toasted almonds, finely chopped

1/8 teaspoon of ground cinnamon

1/2 cup freshly squeezed lemon juice

1 ounce of Parmigiano-Reggiano cheese, finely grated

Instructions

Place the Brussels in a large mixing bowl and place it aside.

Placea non-stick skillet over medium high heat then add the garlic and olive oil. Cook until the garlic turns deep golden brown. Remove from the heat then add the parsley, almonds, cinnamon, and red pepper flakes.

Return the skillet back to the heat sauté for about ten seconds.Remove from the heat, pour in the lemon juice, and then season with salt.

Add the dressing to the Brussels then toss well, add 75% of the cheese, and toss some more. Taste then add the seasoning and top with the rest of the cheese.

Chicken with Pesto

Serves 3 or 4

Ingredients

Water

6 garlic cloves, chopped

Dash of paprika

1 cup of fresh basil leaves

8 cups ofchopped escarole

Salt

1 ounce of Parmigiano-Reggiano cheese, finely grated

Olive oil cooking spray

Dash of cinnamon

Crushed red pepper flakes

1 small onion, thinly sliced

4 cups chicken stock,unsalted

12 ounces of skinless, boneless chicken breast sliced into 1/8 inch thick strips

Instructions

Pour 2 quarts of water in a medium pot and bring to a simmer. You will use this to poach the chicken.

Lightly coat a medium skillet with olive oil cooking spray then place it over medium high heat.

Add the garlic and cook until it turns golden brown. Add the cinnamon, basil leaves, red pepper flakes, onion, and paprika. Cook for roughly 2 minutes until the onion softens.

Add the escarole then cook until it is soft and wilted – for 2 more minutes. Add the stock, bring to a simmer, and then cover. Cook for about 5 minutes or until tender.

Add a pinch of salt to the simmering water and turn off the heat. Add the chicken and stir well until all parts separate. Cook until you notice the strips turning white (meaning they are half cooked). Use a slotted spoon to transfer the strips to a plate to cool.

Let the remaining mixture cook until most of the stock evaporates and looks like thick sauce or soup. Turn off the heat.

Add in half of the cheese, stir, and then season with salt to taste. Add the chicken strips then toss them to coat with the mixture and keep cooking until the strips have cooked enough through, for about 90 seconds.

Top with the remaining cheese, and then serve.

Vegetable Beef Soup

Serves 14

Note: This recipe has many ingredients and it is likely you will hate some vegetables or herbs. You can replace these vegetables and herbs with other ingredients on the negative calorie food list.

Ingredients

4 chopped onions

1 chopped red bell pepper

4 cups of sliced fresh mushrooms

10 chopped celery stalks with their leaves

2 cupsof fresh chopped broccoli

1 small chopped bunch of cilantro

5 box low sodium beef broth

1 large chopped green bell pepper

4 cups of chopped cabbage

6 large chopped fresh carrots

1 finely chopped head of garlic

6 cups of fresh chopped spinach

1 small bunch of Parsley

1 canof asparagus (drained)

2 cans of green beans (drained)

1 cupof canned artichokes (drained)

20 twists of cracked black pepper

1 tablespoon of Italian seasoning

Protein (you can use just about any meat preferably the fishes mentioned in the list)

2 10 oz. cans of tomatoes with green chili's (not drained)

2 cans of diced tomatoes with basil (not drained)

1/2 tablespoon of red pepper flakes

1 tablespoonof dried basil

2 small cans of chopped green chilies (not drained)

1 lb. 80/20 or leaner ground beef (drain if needed)

Instructions

Fill a large cooking pot halfway with the beef, chicken, or vegetable stock. Add all the canned ingredients while draining some as specified intothe pot.

Add water and all the spices then stir. Let it boil for some time, lower the heat to simmer for one hour or until the vegetables soften.

As the soup boils down, add some extra broth and stir.

Serve, garnish as desired, and enjoy.

Snacks

Apple Chips

Serves 2

Ingredients

2 large granny smith apples

1 teaspoon of stevia

1 teaspoon of cinnamon

Canola oil cooking spray

Instructions

Preheat your oven to 200 degrees.

Using a sharp knife, thinlyslice the apples crosswise. Arrange the slices on a single layer on a baking sheet then spray with canola oil cooking spray.

Evenlysprinkle the stevia and cinnamon over the apple slices.

Use the bottom third part of the oven to bake the apples until they are crisp and dry, roughly 2-2½ hours.

Alternatively, you could use a mastrad chipmaker. Not only is it easy and fast, you do not need the cooking spray. Just lay the apple slices on the chipmaker, sprinkle with cinnamon and stevia, and then microwave for 4-5 minutes.

Berry Salad

Serves 4

Ingredients

4 cups of mixed berries (blackberries, raspberries, blueberries, strawberries)

20 whole almonds, toasted and chopped

2 tablespoons of hemp hearts

1/4 cup of cooked quinoa

1 ½ tablespoons of fat free yoghurt

Instructions

Equally divide all the ingredients among four bowls and toss well to mix.

Fruit Salad

Serves 10

Ingredients

2/3 cup of fresh orange juice

1/2 teaspoon of grated lemon zest

2 cups of cubed fresh pineapple

3 kiwi fruits, peeled and sliced

2 oranges, peeled and sectioned

2 cups of blueberries

1/3 cup of fresh lemon juice

1/2 teaspoon of grated orange zest

1 teaspoon of vanilla extract

2 cups of strawberries, hulled and sliced

3 bananas, sliced

1 cup seedless grapes

Instructions

Add orange zest, orange juice, lemon juice and lemon zest, to a saucepan, place it over medium high heat, and bring to boil.

Decrease the heat to medium-low and let it simmer for 5 minutes. Remove from the heat and stir in the vanilla extract. Place it aside to cool.

Place the fruit in a clear glass bowl in layers starting with the pineapple, then strawberries, kiwi, bananas, oranges, then grapes and at the top, blueberries.

Pour the juice over the fruit layers then cover and leave in the fridge for 3-4 hours before serving.

Almond Cake with Berries

Serves 4

Ingredients

½ cup of almond meal

4 packets of monk fruit extract

1 teaspoon of vanilla extract

Olive oil cooking spray

2 eggs, separated; remove 1 yolk

3 tablespoons of raw coconut nectar

Salt

1 cup of mixed berries, mashed well with a fork

Instructions

Preheat your oven to 3750 degrees F.

Bake the almond meal until it becomes aromatic and well toasted –about 3-5 minutes. Remove from the oven and place it on a cool baking sheet.

Place the monk fruit and egg whites in a bowl and whisk until it forms stiff peaks. Use cooking spray to spray four paper cups. Using a toothpick or fork, poke holes in the bottom of each.

Place the almond meal into a mixing bowl then add the egg yolk, salt, vanilla, and coconut nectar. Fold the meringue into the mixture of almond and transfer the batter into the cups.

Place in the microwave and microwave for about thirty seconds. When the mixture has cooked through, place the cups on their sides and give them 45 seconds to cook.

Remove the cakes and place themupside down on four serving plates.

Get them off the cups and serve with berries.

Cucumber and salsa

Serves 2

Ingredients

2 cucumbers, peeled and sliced

12 garlic cloves, minced

¼ cup fresh cilantro, chopped

3 tomatoes, diced

½ sweet onion, diced

Sea salt and black pepper to taste

Instructions

Mix all ingredients except the cucumber in a bowl in order to make the salsa.

Place cucumber slices on a plate and serve with the salsa.

Negative Calorie Diet And Exercise: An Effective Way To Lose Weight Fast

I promised you some unique and cool exercise tips, right? Doing the following exercises will help you burn the fat much faster. All you have to do is to start slow and over time, increase the intensity, keep an open mind, and use the gym (for the ones that require it), where you have an instructor nearby.

Interval Training

This is all about high intensity exercises combined with short periods of rest. This will not only burn more calories than your typical cardio training, it will boost your body's ability to burn fat easily since it increases the production of the growth hormone, which is also a fat burning hormone, and adrenaline which assists in suppressing your appetite.

The intervals will work on your muscles, and help them use oxygen better so that your heart does not have to struggle to pump a lot to make them perform.

Do It!

Get on a treadmill or a stationary bike then use the guide below to start your own interval-training regimen:

Begin with a regular warm-up (any simple exercise to get your blood rushing). When done, run or pedal at a rate that is more than your regular cardio intensity by 20%. If you have never engaged in any serious cardio workouts before, you might want to check this first to understand what I am talking about.

After 30 seconds to 1 minute, reduce the intensity to a rate that is 50% less than the intensity of a regular cardio workout. Alternate the periods of 30 seconds to 1 minute of hard work with 30 seconds to 1 minute of relaxed pedaling or if you want, relaxed running for 6-10 intervals to finish your session.

As this gets simpler, increase each interval's intensity so that you work even longer during the difficult part, reduce your rest periods, or if you feel enthusiastic enough, add more intervals.

Repeat 3-4 times each week.

As you get the hang of this exercise, start the next:

Sprinting

Try sprinting up a hill since the impact on your joints will be much lower and can help you avoid injury. If there is no hilly ground in your area, try the alternative: the dag race approach. Start your sprint by increasing your speed from a jog.

To make the most of this exercise, keep the sprints short – ideally50 yards per sprint. This helps you sustain a high intensity all through and prevents injury.

If you want to increase the overall results of your sprint workout, increase your total number of sprints. This is better than going for long distance runs.

If you are new to exercising, do not do more than one workout per week. You can increase the days once you accustom to the exercise; just remember to allow at least two days of recovery between the workouts.

As you get the hang of the above exercise, start the next:

High Intensity Strength Intervals

Select two exercises that work different muscles completely or ones that use opposite movements. For instance, you can pair a pulling exercise with a pushing exercise or upper body exercise with a lower body exercise like pull-ups and squats.

For the latter, select a weight (if your instructor thinks you need one) with which you can do 10 repetitions. Alternate between the two exercises and do just five repetitions of each move in every set. Remember to rest between the sets so that you finish each set without failing.

Keep alternating between the exercises for a 10 or 15 minutes set time. Keep noting the total number of sets you can do. In subsequent sessions, try to beat your score by completing more sets in the same duration or completing the same number of sets but with heavier weights.

As you get the hang of the above exercises, start the next:

Countdown Workouts

Countdown workouts fit in the use of exercise pairs really well. They also keep you fully engaged in the exercises since you have to keep the count and pay attention.

With every round of the exercise pair, the training encompasses one lesser rep of each move; for instance, you move from a set of six to five...until zero.

You can also try density training where you pair opposing exercises for countdowns. For instance, kettlebell swing, pushups, and squat thrusts would work really well.

Do it!

Start by selecting your pair of exercises.

Perform six repetitions of the first exercise, then six reps of the other move. Go back to the first move and perform five reps then five more of the second exercise. Keep alternating until you reach zero.

In the subsequent workouts, add one rep to each exercise. If you want more countdowns, select a second pair from the list below, or just come up with your own pair of opposing moves.

Squat thrust, pushups

Kettlebell swing, squat thrust

Jumping jacks, pushups

Medicine ball side toss, medicine ball slam

As you get the hang of the above exercise, start the next:

Hurricane Workouts

This is essentially a workout protocol that entails lifting weights and interval training. We have three groups of exercises, called rounds in this type of workouts. Each round has an exercise that increases your heart rate, and a set of other exercises in between.

This design will allow you to keep your heart rate up throughout the workout (and burn significant amounts of calories) that typically lasts 16-22 minutes. Hurricane workouts have five levels and each one is an increased challenge. I have however prepared for you a sample routine you will work with below.

Note: This will require you to be more fit- if fit enough though, you can begin with this:

Warm up for the workout. For all rounds, do one set of each exercise and move on to the next exercise. Finish the whole round thrice before you move to the next round.

First round: Run on a treadmill at 10% incline, 10.5 mph for 25 seconds. Do a kettlebell Turkish getup about 4 times on each side of your body then 10 chin-ups.

Repeat this sequence thrice.

Second round: Run on a treadmill at a 10% incline, 11 mph for 25 seconds. Do 10 dips and a barbell rollout, 15 reps.

Repeat this process thrice.

Third round: Run on a treadmill at a 10% incline, 11.5 mph for 25 seconds. Perform the G.I row, 10 reps. Do the knee grab, 20 reps.

Repeat three times.

I need your help...

Thank you for buying this book!

I hope this book was able to help you to know more about the Negative Calorie Diet and how you can burn fat and lose weight with this diet, the next step is to put what you have learned into practice and actually adopt the diet if you want to see those pounds coming off.

Finally, if you enjoyed this book, then I'd like to ask you for a favor, would you be kind enough to leave a review for this book on Amazon? It'd be greatly appreciated!

I want to reach as many people as I can with this book, and more reviews will help me accomplish that!

If you have any questions or problems, please contact us: hello@freedomdestination.com

Thank you and good luck!

Preview Of '20 Easy And Fast Diet Tips For Losing Weight – An Easy-To-Follow Weight Loss Guide:

Before we start learning about the strategies you can use to lose weight, let's start by highlighting some of the benefits that will come as a result of shedding those extra pounds just to give you extra motivation to want to do something NOW.

Why You Need To Lose Weight

Healthy weight loss has over one hundred benefits; these include emotional and physical benefits. I will dedicate this section to discussing the health benefits that many people (and weight loss/health books) do not pay enough attention to.

1: You Avoid Pre-Diabetes or Type 2 Diabetes

Pre-diabetes/high blood glucose is a condition that develops when the blood sugar levels in your blood move past normal ranges but not enough to qualify as diabetes. When your body stops consistently producing insulin sufficient to meet your body's needs, or the amount produced does not work properly, type 2 diabetes is likely to develop. Being pre-diabetic places you at a very high risk of developing type 2 diabetes.

Being obese or overweight is a proven leading risk factor for type 2 diabetes because carrying excess weight typically makes it hard for cells to respond to insulin, and since the additional fat acts as an insulating layer, it makes it more difficult for the sugar to enter the cells, which results in more circulating blood sugar levels.

Nonetheless, if you are already a pre-diabetic, you can prevent the progression to diabetes by shedding some weight (to reduce the insulating layer on cells so that they respond more to insulin) and trying to maintain a healthy weight.

2: You Keep Your Heart Healthy

When it comes to heart disease, some of the key risk factors are high cholesterol and high blood pressure. Research shows that:

1. Excessive accumulation of body fat makes your body release particular chemicals that occur naturally into the bloodstream, which increases blood pressure, and

2. Being overweight makes the liver produce too much amounts of Low density Lipoprotein (LDL) also called cholesterol. LDL tends to be sticky and gathers in the walls of blood vessels, which causes the narrowing of arteries, a condition called atherosclerosis, which increases your risk of strokes and heart attack.

When you lose weight, your blood pressure often reduces and the liver naturally reduces the amount of LDL it produces.

Royal Adelaide Hospital conducted a research on cardiovascular improvements with respect to a special weight loss program. Their results showed a decrease of cholesterol by 12%, a 10% decrease of LDL, a 5% decrease in diastolic blood pressure, and an 8% decrease in systolic blood pressure.

3: Improved Sleep (and Possible Treatment of Sleep Apnea)

One of the most prominent benefits of losing weight is improved sleep. When you gain excess weight, you gather more soft tissues in the neck; this intensifies the incidence of snoring.

NOTE: Snoring is a result of constricted airways, which obstructs air movement.

Snoring can be a symptom of sleep apnea, a possible life-threatening condition characterized by obstruction of breathing that requires the victim to wake up frequently from sleep to resume breathing.

As a victim of sleep apnea, you rarely remember anything about the episodes of waking many times a night to breathe but even so, this sleep and oxygen deprivation could easily lead to a weak immune system, high blood pressure, heart disease, memory problems, and sexual dysfunction.

When you lose weight, you reduce the amount of fatty tissue in the back of your throat, decrease snoring and the likelihood of the worsening of your health- as aforementioned. You encourage better sleep quality and reduce the risk of developing sleep apnea.

4: Better Joints (Mobile and Pain-Free)

Osteoarthritis (OA) is one of the most common joint disorders. It causes the tissues that protect the joints (cartilage and bone) to wear away. Consequently, the joints become tender and swollen, thus making movement very painful.

When you are overweight, you add to the load placed on the joints that bear the weight such as hips and knees.

NOTE: When you walk, you exert a force of approximately 3-6 times your entire body weight across the knee (read more on this page (check the discussion section) or here), so adding about 10 kg of weight does increase the force on the knees, which is equal to carrying 30-60 kgs² extra.

Therefore, a loss of merely 5% of your body weight could reduce the amount of stress placed on the knees, lower back, and hips, and reduce the pain (remember that losing 5kgs is equal to relieving a force of 15-30kgs² on the knees). According to doctors, a 10% loss of bodyweight has presented a 28% improvement in knee osteoarthritis symptoms.

5: Improved Fertility

There is epidemiological evidence that proves being obese has negative effects on reproduction. There has not been clarity in the mechanisms underlying the relationship between infertility and obesity but research studies suggest that excess body can lead to a serious offset in the metabolism of sex hormones that produce menstrual disruption and consequently, subfertility.

Moreover, when you are pregnant and overweight, you a more likely to miscarry and (or) develop other medical complications, and in particular, gestational diabetes, pregnancy induced hypertension, thromboembolism, and preeclampsia. There are reports to show that deliveries in obese women show increased rates of labor induction, caesarian section, and problematic labor caused by increased size of the unborn baby.

Additionally, experts report that a baby of an overweight woman is more likely to require more medical attention (admission to neonatal intensive care) and develop congenital defects such as cardiac and neural tube problems.

Moreover, obese individuals are more likely to experience birth related injuries and the likelihood of giving birth to babies with large birth weights, which puts them at risk of birth trauma and a possibility of childhood and probably lifelong obesity. Reducing weight in this case could help you and your baby avoid all these health problems.

Emotional Weight Loss Benefits

The negativity usually around overweight people affects your self-esteem and confidence. Naturally, when you are carrying some excess weight, you will worry about how other people see you and become overly anxious in particular situations. This affects many aspects of your life including your job interactions and performance, school, and your life at home (in the neighborhood).

Losing weight will help you gain confidence and increase your self-worth and self-love; losing weight normally makes you cheerful and as a result, your relationships with other people improve. Most of your fears and anxieties related to being overweight disappear and in general, you live a better life.

Once you regain your confidence, you feel in control. This becomes the status quo once you become comfortable with your new weight. Once you lose the weight, you are more comfortable when making food related decisions.

You also feel and become more honest when you interact with others and can better articulate your thoughts and feelings. You will no longer hold back since you are more self-possessed about your appearance and health.

Now that you know some of the benefits you stand to gain from losing weight, let us discuss the various effortless ways to lose weight.

Check out the rest of 20 Easy And Fast Diet Tips For Losing Weight on Amazon, go to:**http://amzn.to/2oI1Kyx**

Check Out My Other Books

Below you'll find some of my other popular books that are popular on Amazon and Kindle as well.

Alternatively, you can visit my author page on Amazon to see other work done by me.

20 Easy And Fast Diet Tips For Losing Weight – An Easy-To-Follow Weight Loss Guide

Belly Diet: The Zero Belly Diet Step-By-Step Guide Which Will Help You To Lose Your Belly And Enjoy Your Flat Belly

Anti-Inflammatory Diet Guide – The Guide To Reduce Inflammation And Live A Healthy Life Without Pain

Dash Diet: Cookbook For Weight Loss With Action Plan And Easy Recipes

Clean Eating: Cookbook And Guide To Restore Your Body's Natural Balance And Eat Healthy

Negative Calorie Diet: Cookbook & Guide Which Help You To Burn Body Fat, Lose Weight And Live Healthy

Smart Fat: Cookbook With Fat Meals Which Help You To Lose Weight, Get Healthy And Improve Brain Function

Smart Fat

Cookbook With Fat Meals Which Help You To Lose Weight, Get Healthy And Improve Brain Function

LELA GIBSON

INTRODUCTION

I want to thank you and congratulate you for buying the book, *"Smart Fat"*.

This book contains proven steps and strategies on how to use fat meals to lose weight, get healthy and improve brain function.

For many years, fat has held a bad reputation. Many blamed it for weight gain and various diseases, including stroke and heart attack. Recent research, however, shows that it does not matter that you eat fat- it matters that you eat the right kind of fat. There are many proven benefits to eating the right kinds of fat, often monounsaturated, polyunsaturated, and Omega-3s. These benefits include:

- Increased satiety, meaning less hunger cravings and improved weight loss or maintenance efforts

- Decreased LDL levels, which lowers the risk of heart disease and stroke

- Improved energy levels, especially when the right fats are paired with a low-carb diet

- Better absorption of fat-soluble vitamins like A, D, E, and K

- Improved brain function from encouraging the production of cell membranes in the brain

This book is filled with recipes that rely on smart fat, the fat that is going to offer all the above benefits. Whether you are eating for your health, to improve brain function, or to lose weight, best of luck with your goals!

Thanks again for buying this book, I hope you enjoy it!

CONTENTS

How To Increase Fat In Your Diet

The fat diet sounds easy but it can be difficult to implement. This is because it's not easy to go against the grain. For years, fat has been the bad guy. Therefore, it may take a bit of effort to change that mentality. However, don't worry because you can take a number of different steps to increase your fat intake like:

Ease into fat consumption

No matter how great the fat diet is for you, you may end up abandoning it within a few days if you rush into it. This is because your body is not used to burning fat. It needs time to adjust. This is especially so if you are used to eating high carb foods and sugary snacks.

Therefore, take it slow. Give yourself room to grow into the diet. You can start by slowly increasing your fat consumption even as you decrease the consumption of high carb foods. Here's the thing. Your body needs fuel in order to function. It can easily get this fuel from carbohydrates. However, if you decrease your consumption of high carb foods, your body will adapt to burning fat for fuel.

Gradually increasing the amount of fat you eat will enable you to adjust to the fat diet. Once you adapt to it, you'll have no issue burning fat. In addition, your palate will also adjust to eating the 'rich' high fat foods.

Top and garnish with fat

A great way to increase fat in your diet is by using every opportunity to add it to you foods. The first thing you need to do is cook with oil. Forget about boiling or steaming your food. Instead, fry it in fat.

Next, drizzle your food with oil. Foods such as salads and flourless gravy taste better with a dollop of oil. You can even add oil to things such as sour cream, butter and mayo. The important thing is to top your food with fat. The same goes for garnishing. If you want to add garnish, go for high fat foods such as nuts, seeds, olives, avocado and cheese. These toppings can be added to various dishes. Thus, you should take advantage of them.

While we're at it, don't forget to snack on fat if you feel hungry in between meals. You can eat foods such as boiled eggs, cheese and nuts. This will keep you satisfied as you wait for your next meal. In addition, such foods will not mess up your diet.

Experiment with different types of fat

One thing you need to know about food is that various ingredients can make a difference to the way a certain meal tastes. For example, eggs fried with butter taste different from ones cooked with olive oil. This means you can have fun experimenting on the fat diet. You can switch up fats such as avocado oil, coconut oil, butter, sesame oil, olive oil, almond oil, macadamia oil and walnut oil whenever you try out certain recipes. You can also experiment with lard, duck fat and tallow. This will allow you to discover different tastes and keep things fresh.

Overall, the fat diet is not meant to be difficult to follow or boring. You can have fun with it if you give your body time to adjust and if you allow yourself to experiment with various types of fat. So go on, try it.

In the following chapters, we will look at various recipes you can try out while the fat diet.

Breakfast Recipes

Coconut-Raisin Quinoa

Quinoa is a food that can be sweet or savory. In this dish, plump raisins and coconut make it sweet while lime zest and cilantro add a savory touch. A dressing keeps the quinoa moist and tender.

Ingredients (for 4 servings)

For the quinoa:

- 1 cup quinoa (well rinsed)

- ¼ cup raisins

- ¼ cup unsweetened coconut

- 1 ¾ cups water

- 1 tablespoon coconut oil

- ¼ cup cilantro (minced)

- Zest of one lime

For the dressing:

- 2 tablespoons grape seed oil (or canola oil)

- 2 tablespoons lime juice

- ¾ teaspoon honey

- ¼ teaspoon salt

- Pinch of pepper

Instructions

Add the coconut oil to a small pot over medium heat. When warmed, at the quinoa and allow it to toast for 3-4 minutes, until it begins to stick to the pot. Then, the added water and salt to the pot and turn up the heat. Bring the quinoa to a boil and then set to a simmer, cooking for about 20 minutes until the quinoa is fluffy and the liquid is absorbed.

Use a fork to fluff the quinoa and then mix in the coconut flakes and lime zest. Partially cover the quinoa and allow it to sit an additional 10 minutes before transferring to a bowl. Set the bowl at room temperature until cooled.

While you are waiting, whisk the ingredients for the dressing together in a small bowl. You may want to warm the honey slightly if you cannot get it to mix well with the other ingredients. Once cooled, stir in the raisins and cilantro. Drizzle with the dressing and toss to combine.

Barley with Sunflower Seeds and Bananas

This filling breakfast option combines sweet and nutty flavors. The sunflower seeds provide plenty of healthy fat. Since you can make it in the microwave, it is a quick breakfast option that does not skimp on flavor. If you want a softer barley, consider soaking it the night before.

Ingredients (for 2 servings)

- 2/3 cup pearl barley (quick cooking)

- 1 1/3 cups water

- ¼ cup unsalted sunflower seeds

- 2 medium bananas (sliced)

- 2 teaspoons honey

Instructions

Add the barley and water to a bowl and cook in the microwave on high heat for about 6 minutes, or until done. You may need to adjust this time based on your microwave. Stir the barley and allow it to sit for 2 minutes. When you are ready to eat, top with the sunflower seeds, sliced bananas, and honey.

Cheesy Bacon Quiche

This simple quiche is light, fluffy, and high in the right kinds of fat. A prepared piecrust makes this quick and easy to throw together. You also save time if you use a can of real bacon bits instead of waiting for your bacon to cook before preparing the quiche.

Ingredients (for 6 servings)

- 1 9-inch pie crust (deep dish, unthawed)

- 1 can (3 ounces) real bacon bits

- 1 cup half-and-half

- 4 eggs (lightly beaten)

- ¾ cup Swiss cheese (shredded)

- ¼ cup Parmesan cheese (grated)

- 1 medium onion (chopped)

Instructions

Set the oven to 400 degrees so it can preheat. While you are waiting, add both cheeses, the bacon bits, and the chopped onions to a bowl and mix together. Then, transfer this into the piecrust.

Add the eggs and half-and-half to another bowl and mix together to incorporate. Pour this into the piecrust, covering the bacon-cheese mixture.

Place your prepared quiche in the oven for 15 minutes. Then, reduce the temperature to 350 degrees for 35 more minutes, until the eggs have set and the top of the quiche starts to brown.

Banana Walnut Pancakes

These pancakes have all the deliciousness of banana-nut bread in an easier, breakfast friendly form. They are also a great way to use up your softening bananas before they go bad.

Ingredients (for 3 servings)

- 1 large or 2 small bananas (overripe)

- ¼ cup walnuts (finely chopped)

- 1 cup all-purpose flour)

- 1 egg

- 1 cup almond milk

- 3 tablespoons granulated sugar

- 1 ½ tablespoons butter (melted)

- 1 tablespoon baking powder

- ½ teaspoon baking soda

- ½ teaspoon cinnamon

- ½ teaspoon nutmeg

- ½ teaspoon vanilla extract

- ½ teaspoon salt

Instructions

Add the walnuts, flour, sugar, baking soda and powder, cinnamon, nutmeg, and salt to a large bowl and mix together to incorporate. Then, make a well in the center of the dry mixture.

In a separate bowl, mash the banana. Then, whisk in the melted butter, almond milk, and vanilla extract. Once smooth, whisk in the egg. Pour this into the well you made in the flour mixture and stir to combine, being careful not to over mix.

Add olive oil or cooking spray to a skillet over medium-high heat. Use about ¼ cup of batter to make each pancake. Drop the batter in and tilt the skillet slightly, carefully spreading it around. Cook about 3-4 minutes until the edges become firm and bubbles start to form. Then, flip and cook an additional 2-3 minutes on the other side.

Easy Baked Egg and Avocado Breakfast Bowl

This is a simple, but flavorful recipe. You can serve as recommended in this recipe, or tweak it by adding some of your favorite flavors.

Ingredients (for 4 servings)

- 8 eggs

- 4 avocados

- 4 flour or corn tortillas (warmed)

- 2 limes

- 1 teaspoon salt

- ½ teaspoon black pepper

- Scallions (optional, sliced for serving)

- Cilantro (optional, chopped for serving)

- Chilies (optional, sliced for serving)

Instructions

Start by preheating the oven to 450 degrees. Use a sharp knife to cut each avocado in half, carefully removing the pit. Take a spoon and remove about 1 ½ tablespoons of flesh from the avocado, so the opening is large enough that the egg fits in. Cut the limes in half and squeeze each over 2 of the avocado halves, coating with flesh. Sprinkle salt on top and place on a baking tray.

Once all the avocado halves are prepared, break one egg into each. Season with salt and pepper to taste. Be sure to keep the yolk intact, even if some of the white spills over. If you want your avocados presented nicely, consider using a sieve to separate some of the egg white before putting it inside the avocado.

Cook in the preheated oven for 10-12 minutes, until the yolk is runny but the whites are set. Garnish with the toppings and serve with the warmed tortillas.

Lunch Recipes

Mexican-Inspired Salmon Cilantro Burgers

This salmon patty is much tastier than ground beef and topped with a cilantro-lime mayo that gives it a Southwest kick. Eat this burger alone for lunch or pair with a side for a filling dinner.

Ingredients (for 8 servings)

- 2 pounds salmon fillet (with skin removed and cut into 1-inch pieces)

- ½ cup dry breadcrumbs

- ½ cup canola mayonnaise

- 1 green onion (chopped)

- ¼ cup + 2 tablespoons cilantro (chopped)

- 1 small jalapeno pepper (seeded and minced)

- ¼ cup + 2 tablespoons fresh lime juice

- 1 teaspoon + ½ teaspoon salt

- ½ teaspoon + ¼ teaspoon pepper

- Cooking spray

Optional for topping:

- Sesame seed hamburger buns

- Lettuce leaves (1 per burger)

- English cucumber slices (3 per burger)

Instructions

Add the mayonnaise, 2 tablespoons of lime juice, 2 tablespoons of cilantro, and ¼ teaspoon each of salt and pepper to a small bowl and whisk to combine. Set this in the fridge to chill while you prepare the burgers.

Add the salmon chunks to a food processor and pulse until it is coarsely chopped. Then, add the remaining ingredients to the processor and pulse until well combined. Form this into 8 patties.

Place a grill pan on the stove and warm it to medium-high heat. Use cooking spray to coat the pan before adding the patties. Cook about 2 minutes on each side, until cooked to your desired level of doneness. Serve the salmon with the mayonnaise mixture on a bun, topping with the lettuce and English cucumbers if you choose.

Crab Cakes

These flavorful patties can be enjoyed as a standalone, as a slider, or as a side to a salad. They make for an easy and delicious lunch and even taste good reheated, so you can make them a couple days ahead of time and grab them for your lunch or a snack throughout the day.

Ingredients (for 8 servings)

- 1 pound fresh lump crab meat

- 1 can pink salmon (boneless, skinless)

- 3 eggs

- ½ cup pork rinds (crushed)

- 2 tablespoons mayo

- 2 tablespoons avocado flesh

- 1 tablespoon lemon juice

- 1 tablespoon garlic powder

- 1 tablespoon relish

- 1 teaspoon salt

- Olive oil for frying

Instructions

Add everything except the olive oil to a large bowl and mix to combine. Be cautious of over mixing. Form this into 8 patties and set to the side.

Set a skillet on the stove over medium heat. Add the olive oil and allow to warm before adding the patties, 2 at a time. Cook for about 6 minutes on each side, until the patties are golden brown.

Seared Chicken Breast Halves and Strawberry Avocado Salsa

This dish tastes great on top of the salad and is perfect when strawberries are in season. The recipe does call for jalapeno, which gives this dish a small kick but not much. You can omit them if you choose.

Ingredients (for 4 servings)

- 4 chicken breast halves (about 4 ounces each)

- 1 medium avocado (diced)

- 1 ½ cups strawberries (chopped)

- 2 tablespoons cilantro (chopped)

- 2 tablespoons jalapeno pepper (seeded and minced)

- 1 tablespoon olive oil

- 2 teaspoons lime juice

- ½ teaspoon + ¼ teaspoon salt

- ¼ teaspoon pepper

- 1 lime (cut into 4 wedges, for serving)

Instructions

Add the avocado, strawberries, jalapeno, lime juice, cilantro, and ¼ teaspoon of the salt to a small bowl. Gently but thoroughly mix to combine. Set this to the side.

Place a large skillet on the stove and warm to medium heat. Add the oil and allow it to warm before distributing it around the pan. Then, pat the chicken dry with paper towels and add the remaining salt and the pepper to both sides of each breast. Cook the chicken for about 4-5 minutes on one side and then flip, cooking an additional 4-5 minutes. Cook longer if necessary so the chicken is cooked all the way through.

If you are serving as a salad, prepare the lettuce on the plates. Add one chicken breast half to each plate and top with the strawberry avocado salsa. Garnish with a lime wedge.

Open-Faced Avocado and Salmon BLT

Tender, flaky salmon and creamy avocado top this traditional BLT on a single slice of toasted bread. Creamy, flaky, and crispy ingredients will excite your taste buds. Plus, who doesn't love bacon?

Ingredients (for 4 servings)

- 4 salmon fillets (3/4" thick, about 4 ounces)- with skin removed

- 4 slices rustic Italian bread

- 4 slices center-cut bacon

- ½ avocado (peeled and pitted, cut into 8 slices)

- 4 tomato slices (1/4-inch thick)

- 4 lettuce leaves

- ¼ cup canola mayo

- 1 ½ teaspoons Dijon mustard

- 2 tablespoons water

- 2 teaspoons + 1 teaspoon fresh chives (minced)

- ½ lemon (cut into 4 wedges, for garnish)

Instructions

Set the broiler on high heat. When heated, place the Italian bread on a baking sheet and broil until toasted, flipping the bread half way through so both sides are browned. This should take about 1 minute on each side.

Then, place the bacon in a nonstick skillet and cook over medium heat. Once crispy, remove it from the pan and set to the side on a rack or a plate with a paper towel. Put the salmon in the pan you cooked the bacon in and cook 8 minutes total, flipping halfway through. You can adjust this cooking time to your desired doneness.

While you are waiting for the salmon to finish cooking, add the mayo, Dijon mustard, water, and 2 teaspoons of the chives to a small bowl and mix thoroughly to incorporate. Spread this mixture on the toasted bread. Then, assemble the sandwiches by adding 1 leaf of lettuce, 1 tomato slice, 1 bacon slice, 1 fish fillet, and 2 slices of avocado to each piece of bread. Sprinkle with the remaining chives and garnish with lemon wedges for serving.

Dinner

Salmon with Toasted Walnuts and Walnut Sherry Vinaigrette

Healthy fats in this recipe come from walnuts, walnut oil, and omega-3 rich salmon. This can be served over a bed of asparagus, snap peas, or cauliflower rice. It also tastes great on top of a salad.

Ingredients (for 4 servings)

- 4 boneless salmon fillets with skin on (about 1/3 pound each)

- ½ cup toasted walnut halves (chopped)

- 1/3 cup shallots (diced)

- 1/3 cup walnut oil

- ¼ cup Sherry vinegar

- 1 tablespoon olive oil

- 1 teaspoon sugar

- Salt and pepper to taste

Instructions

Set the oven to 375 degrees so it can preheat. Place a 9x13 roasting pan until it preheats (do not use glass). While you are waiting, place the salmon with the skin side down on a plate or cutting board and add salt and pepper to taste. Carefully remove the roasting pan and place the salmon skin side down inside of it.

Bake the salmon for 8-10 minutes, until it flakes with a fork. You want to be very careful not to overcook it, because it will become dry very fast.

While you are waiting, place a small skillet on the stove over medium heat. Add the shallots and cook until golden in color and softened, for about 2 minutes. Then, add the sugar and stir until it dissolves. Once dissolved, add the vinegar and some salt and pepper. Cook an additional minute before removing from the stove.

Add the oil and shallot mixture to a medium bowl. Add the walnut oil and whisk until well combined. Then, stir in the walnuts. Once the salmon is cooked, add to a plate and drizzle with the vinaigrette. Serve with your chosen side.

Dinner

Single-Skillet Seared Avocado and Chicken

Robust, hearty flavors come together in this dish that won't leave every pan in your home dirty. A small amount of sugar is used while searing the avocados to char them and bring out their flavors.

Ingredients (for 4 servings)

- 4 boneless, skinless chicken breast halves (about 6 ounces each)

- 4 green onions (trimmed)

- 2 small ripened avocados (cut in half with pits removed)

- 1/3 cup sour cream

- 2 medium red onions (cut into ¼" rings)

- 1 poblano pepper (sliced)

- 3 tablespoons lime juice

- 2 tablespoons water

- 1 tablespoon soy sauce

- 1 tablespoon olive oil

- ¼ teaspoon + ¼ teaspoon sea salt

- ½ teaspoon ancho chili powder

- ½ teaspoon black pepper

- ¼ teaspoon sugar

- 1 lime (cut into 4 wedges, for garnish)

- 8 sprigs cilantro (for garnish)

Instructions

Set the oven to 450 degrees so it can preheat. Set a large cast iron skillet on the stove and warm to a medium-high temperature. Place the olive oil inside and distribute evenly.

While you are waiting for the olive oil to warm, add the chili powder, pepper, and ¼ teaspoon salt to the chicken. Add to the pan and cook for 4 minutes. Then, flip it and cook another minute. Transfer to a plate (it will not be fully cooked yet).

Carefully wipe the skillet with paper towels to clean it. Add a non-stick cooking spray and turn up the temperature to high heat. Sprinkle the sugar on top of the avocado halves and place them cut side down in the pan. Cook until charred, about 2 minutes. Remove from the skillet and set aside.

Then, spray the pan again and add the red onions. Char on high heat for about 3 minutes and flip, adding the poblano pepper and green onions. Use a fork to separate the rings of the onion and toss with the green onions and poblano. Stir the soy sauce and lime juice into the pan and distribute.

Distribute the chicken breast halves and avocados across the pan and bake for about 7 minutes in the oven, until the chicken is cooked all the way through.

When the chicken is cooked, remove from the oven and let cool slightly. While you are waiting, mix together the sour cream and water in a bowl. Serve the chicken and avocados with the sour cream mixture and top with a lime wedge and 2 sprigs of cilantro each. Sprinkle with remaining salt if you would like.

Crockpot Thai Pork and Peppers with Peanut Sauce

Using a quality nut butter is important to get the healthy fats from this recipe. The peanut sauce and tender pork pairs beautifully. It is even better that this is a low-maintenance crockpot meal that you can throw together and then forget about for a few hours. If you gather the ingredients ahead of time, it takes less time to prepare this than to call for Thai takeout.

Ingredients (for 4 servings)

- 1 pound boneless pork chops

- 2 red bell peppers (cut into thin slices, then into bite-sized pieces)

- 6 cloves garlic (minced)

- 1 cup low-sodium chicken broth

- 1/3 cup creamy nut butter

- 1/3 cup soy sauce

- 3 tablespoons honey

- 2 tablespoons ginger (minced)

- 1 teaspoon red pepper flakes

Instructions

Add all the ingredients except the pork chops in the slow cooker and stir to combine. Then, place the pork chops inside and spoon the mixture over them, coating thoroughly. Cook for 5-6 hours on the low heat setting of your crock pot.

Once the pork is tender, carefully remove it from the pot and place it on a cutting board. Use two forks to shred the pork into pieces. Then, return the pork to the crock pot and stir into the sauce. Allow to cook an additional 10-15 minutes while the pork soaks up more of the peanut sauce and serve. You can eat this alone, with a side of white, brown, or cauliflower rice, or with a side of veggies.

Bacon and Cheese Stuffed Chicken Breasts with Lemony Green Beans and Almonds

Tender chicken breasts are filled with goat's cheese and bacon for a salty, creamy experience. The green beans with almonds have a nice, bright flavor in comparison.

Ingredients (for 2 servings)

For the chicken:

- 2 chicken breasts (with or without skin)

- ¾ cup goats cheese (softened to room temperature)

- 2 slices bacon (chopped)

- 1 tablespoon olive oil

- ½ teaspoon salt

- ¼ teaspoon pepper

For the green beans:

- 1 cup green beans (cleaned and trimmed)

- Juice of ½ lemon

- Zest of ½ lemon

- ¼ cup almonds (toasted and chopped)

Instructions

Add the bacon to a medium skillet and fry until lightly golden in color. Then, carefully remove the bacon with a slotted spoon and place on a plate lined with a paper towel.

Place the chicken breasts on a cutting board and pat dry with a paper towel. Season them with the salt and pepper and then use a sharp knife to cut down the middle on one side, keeping the inside sealed.

Take the cooled bacon and put it in the bowl with the goats cheese. Mix until incorporated and add extra pepper if you would like. Then, stuff the breasts with this mixture and gently close. You can use a toothpick if you would like.

Bring the olive oil to temperature over medium high heat and add the chicken breasts to the skillet. Cook until the chicken is cooked completely and golden brown, about 4-5 minutes on each side. Set this to the side to rest while you prepare the green beans.

Bring water and a little salt to a boil and put the green beans in the pan for 1-2 minutes. Rinse them with cool water and then drizzle with the lemon juice. Top with the toasted almonds and lemon zest and serve alongside the chicken.

Miso Salmon and Wilted Spinach

This Asian-inspired dish tastes great on top of rice, either white or brown. If you want a lower carb option, you could try cauliflower rice as well.

Ingredients (for 2 servings)

For the fish:

- 2 salmon fillets (about 6 ounces, with skin removed)

- 1 tablespoon white miso paste

- 2 teaspoons low-sodium soy sauce

- 2 teaspoons rice vinegar

- 2 teaspoons sweet rice wine (mirin)

- 1 teaspoon toasted sesame seeds

- ½ teaspoon fresh ginger (grated)

- ½ teaspoon sugar

For the wilted spinach:

- 10 ounces (1 package) fresh spinach

- 1 teaspoon minced garlic

- 2 teaspoons low-sodium soy sauce

- 2 teaspoons dark sesame oil

Instructions

Turn on the broiler so it can preheat. Add all the ingredients for the fish except the salmon and sesame seeds to a small bowl. Whisk to incorporate and set to the side.

Prepare a baking tray by lining it with foil. Use a brush to paint the prepared miso mixture on each fillet, making a thick and even coating. Place these in the broiler for about 8 minutes, or until the fish reaches your desired doneness level. When it is done, sprinkle with the toasted sesame seeds before serving.

A couple minutes before the salmon is done, warm the sesame oil to medium-high heat in a large skillet. Add the spinach and garlic and cook until the spinach just starts to wilt, about 30 seconds as you continuously toss the mixture. Then, stir in the soy sauce and remove from heat. Serve alongside the salmon fillets.

Soup, Side, and Snack Recipes

Tortilla Soup with Avocado and Shrimp

The healthy fats in this delicious soup come from the shrimp and the avocado. It has the perfect blend of smokiness and spiciness to delight your taste buds. You can garnish with cheddar, sour cream, or cilantro in addition to the tortilla strips.

Ingredients (for 4 servings)

- 12 ounces medium-sized shrimp (peeled and deveined, with tails removed)

- 1 cup avocado (diced)

- 4 cups low-sodium chicken broth

- 1 can (15 ounces) fire-roasted diced tomatoes (with juices)

- 1 can (15 ounces) white hominy (drained and rinsed)

- 1 ounce tortilla chips (lightly crushed)

- 1 cup onion (chopped)

- 1/3 cup carrot (chopped)

- 1/3 cup celery (chopped)

- 3 garlic cloves (minced)

- 1 tablespoon chipotle chili in adobo sauce (minced)

- 1 tablespoon lime juice

- 1 tablespoon olive oil

- 1 teaspoon chili powder

- 1 teaspoon cumin

Instructions

Place a Dutch oven or a large soup pot on the stove and warm to medium-high heat. Add the olive oil and distribute. Then, add the onion, carrot, celery, garlic, chipotle chili, chili powder, and cumin to the pan. Stir until the carrot starts to become tender, about 6 minutes. Then, add the fire-roasted tomatoes, hominy, and chicken broth. Turn up the heat and bring the mixture to a boil.

Once boiling, cover the pot and cook for 6 minutes. Then, add the shrimp and cook all the way through, about 2 minutes. Take the pan off the stove and add the salt and lime juice. Stir to incorporate. Serve in bowls and top with the avocado and crushed chips, as well as any other toppings you choose.

Apple Walnut Salad

This sweet and savory salad offers a medley of flavors and a medley of healthy fats. Its fat sources include walnuts, cream cheese, and full-fat yogurt. This tastes great alongside chicken or pork and is so tasty you could eat it alone for dessert.

Ingredients (for 8 servings)

- 6 large apples (cored, peeled, and diced)

- 1 ½ cups + ¼ cup walnuts (chopped)

- 1 container (6 ounces) full-fat plain yogurt

- 1 package (8 ounces) cream cheese (softened)

- 1 cup dried cranberries

- ¾ cup brown sugar

- 1 teaspoon vanilla

- 1 teaspoon cinnamon

Instructions

Mix the brown sugar and cinnamon together in a bowl. Then, add the yogurt, cream cheese, and vanilla and beat until smooth. Stir in the chopped apples, dried cranberries, and 1 ½ cups of walnuts. Mix until everything is thoroughly coated. Place in a bowl and top with the remaining walnuts. Chill 1-2 hours before serving.

Avocado Citrus Salad

This citrus-y salad makes the perfect pairing with chicken, pork, or even fish that is rich in healthy fats. It can also be eaten as a standalone lunch or snack.

Ingredients (for 4 servings)

- 2 avocados (halved, pitted, peeled, and cut into slices)

- 1 large pink grapefruit

- 1 head romaine lettuce

- 2 tablespoons white wine vinegar

- 4 tablespoons olive oil

- 1 teaspoon salt

- ½ teaspoon pepper

Instructions

Take a paring knife (or a zester) and remove 1 tablespoon of zest from the grapefruit, being sure to avoid the white bitter-tasting pith found under the peel. Then, use a sharp knife to cut the grapefruit in half over a medium bowl. Cut into the individual segments of grapefruit by slicing along the membrane on either side, leaving behind the membrane as you work. Set the bowl to the side and reserve the grapefruit rind halves.

Take the vinegar, oil, and salt and pepper and add it to a medium bowl. Whisk it together and then squeeze the grapefruit rinds over the bowl, extracting the remaining juice. Stir in the zest.

Next, put the avocado slices in the bowl and coat with the dressing, spooning it over gently so the avocados remain intact. Gently stir in the grapefruit segments you set to the side. Set this bowl to the side while you roughly chop the romaine lettuce into bite-sized pieces. Serve this on four individual plates and top each with ¼ of the grapefruit and avocado slices and drizzle with the remaining dressing.

White Bean Salad with Bacon, Cheddar, and Walnuts

This savory salad makes a perfect accompaniment to fish, chicken, or pork. It offers healthy fats from the cheddar cheese and walnuts.

Ingredients (for 10 servings)

- 3 can (15 ounces each) white Great Northern beans (drained and rinsed)

- 4 slices bacon (cooked, cooled, and crumbled)

- 1 medium red bell pepper (minced)

- 2 whole garlic heads

- ½ cup sharp cheddar cheese (shredded)

- ½ cup toasted walnuts (chopped)

- ½ cup parsley (chopped)

- ½ cup celery (chopped)

- 1/3 cup + 1 teaspoon olive oil

- 2 tablespoons apple cider vinegar

- 1 tablespoon Dijon mustard

- 1 teaspoon salt

- ½ teaspoon pepper

Instructions

Start by setting the oven to 350 degrees to preheat. Carefully remove the extra skin layers from the garlic, without separating the individual cloves. Then, slice the tips off and set the garlic on a piece of foil. Use the single teaspoon of oil to drizzle the heads and wrap them in the foil. Cook until slightly browned and soft, about an hour. Once the garlic is finished, carefully unwrap it and set it to the side to cool.

When cooled, squeeze the cloves out of their skins and into a food processor. Then, add the remaining oil, along with the mustard, vinegar, and thyme. Puree until smooth before adding the salt and pepper. Then, pulse to combine.

Next, add the beans to a large bowl with the crumbled bacon, toasted walnuts, bell pepper, parsley, and celery. Mix to combine and coat with the dressing. Then, add the cheese and gently stir. You can chill before serving or eat at room temperature.

Healthy Fat Olive Balls

These balls have olives, cream cheese, and pecans, all of which are great sources of healthy fats. These little bites are great for an anytime snack and even work well as an appetizer for parties.

Ingredients (for 25 servings)

- ½ jar (3.5 ounces) green olives (with pimentos)

- 2 tablespoons juice from the olives

- ¾ cup pecans (chopped)

- 1 package (8 ounces) cream cheese (softened)

- ¼ teaspoon seasoned salt

Instructions

Add the cream cheese, seasoned salt, and 2 tablespoons olive juice to a food processor and pulse until well combined. Transfer to a bowl and place in the refrigerator for about 30 minutes, until it firms.

Once firm, use the mixture to surround each olive. You should have enough mixture to make 12-13 balls. Place the pecans in a shallow bowl or on a plate and roll the balls in them. Place them on a wax-lined tray and return to the refrigerator to firm up. You can then cut in halves if you would like- each ball is 2 servings.

Buttermilk Avocado Soup Topped with Crab Salad

Crab is a good source of Omega-3s and avocados are rich in monounsaturated fats. You can adjust the amount of buttermilk added until your soup achieves a smooth, creamy consistency. This will also cut down on some of the avocado flavor, if you do not want a strong avocado taste.

Ingredients (for 8 servings)

For the soup:

- 4 ripened avocados (pitted and peeled)

- 1 ½ cups fat-free buttermilk

- 2 small tomatillos (chopped)

- ½ cup low-sodium chicken broth

- 1 large clove garlic

- 2 serrano peppers (seeded)

- 3/4 teaspoon salt

For the crab salad:

- 16 ounces crab meat (drained)

- ¼ cup red bell pepper (minced)

- 2 tablespoons chives (chopped)

- 1 tablespoon lemon juice

- 1 teaspoon orange zest

Instructions

Add all the ingredients for the soup to a blender. Blend until you have a smooth, creamy consistency. Adjust the buttermilk as needed to meet your preference.

Then, add the crab and other ingredients to a large bowl. Gently toss everything until well combined. Serve the soup in a bowl with the crab salad on top.

I need your help...

Thank you again for buying this book!

I hope this book was able to help you to get an idea about how to use fat meals to lose weight, get healthy and improve brain function.

The next step is to take action.

Finally, if you enjoyed this book, then I'd like to ask you for a favor, would you be kind enough to leave a review for this book on Amazon? It'd be greatly appreciated!

I want to reach as many people as I can with this book, and more reviews will help me accomplish that!

If you have any questions or problems, please contact us: hello@freedomdestination.com

Thank you and good luck!